No More Cavities

Brian Cusp

No More Cavities

Brian Cusp

In Search of Better Dental
Health
ISBN-13: 978-1979559201

Warning

Do not use any of these products

or treatments in this book without

first consulting your dentist

and doctor.

Table of Contents

Chapter One - What is a Cavity?

Tooth decay is caused by particles of food left on the teeth particularly foods containing sugars and starches. Bacteria in the mouth feed on these foods producing acids that eat away at the tooth enamel causing decay.

Experts say that deficiency of calcium, magnesium, and phosphorus, and lack of soluble vitamins especially Vitamin D, and use of processed sugar are major contributing factors in causing cavities.

Plaque on the teeth is a major problem. It is a sticky film that builds up on your teeth and contains millions of bacteria, causing both tooth decay and gum disease.

Cavities are caused by tooth demineralization which is caused by a pH in the mouth of 5.5 pH and below. The mouth is normally 7.0, neutral acidity. Saliva is 7.0 acidity. Acidic foods and acidic drinks lower the pH in the mouth particularly sugar as it clings to the teeth and bacteria feed on the sugar creating acids making the mouth more acidic.

Chapter Two - What is pH?

PH is a numeric scale to specify Acidity or Basicity. The range is from zero to fourteen on a logarithmic scale. Seven is neutral, and water is neutral with a pH of 7. Hydrochloric Acid is zero, Stomach Acid is one, Lemon Juice is two, Orange Juice is 3.3 to 4.2, Beer and Cola are three, Saliva is 7.1 to 7.5, Milk is 6.5 to 6.7, ordinary Yoghurt is 4.5 to 4.7, the gastric acid in Stomach is 1.3 to 3.5, Apples 3.3, Beets 5.3 to 6.3, Honey Dew Melon 6.3, Maple Syrup 5.15, Various Sugars around 7.0, Bread 5.0 to 6.2, Butter 6.2, Hamburger 6.2, Egg White 8.2, Egg Yolk 6.6, Ham 5.5, Blood pH should be 7.4 to be healthy, Vinegar 2.4, Flounder 6.4 to 6.9, Overall Fish is rated acidic, Coffee 5, Mouthwashes range from 4.6 to 6.5, Fluoride is 6.6,

Whitening Tooth Products average 8.2, Baking Soda (Sodium Bicarbonate) is 8.3, Whitening Tooth Products average 6.3, Whitening Toothpastes average 6.3, and Chicken Breasts 5.6 to 6.4, Chocolate 6.5, Green Beans 5.1 – 5.6, Onions 5.5 – 6.5, Potatoes 4.8 to 5.4, Ice Cream 6.5 to 7.0, Tomato Juice 4.45, Broccoli and Brussel Sprouts and Cabbage 6.5, Lettuce 6.0 to 7.0, and Rice is 6.0 to 6.7.

A pH lower than 7 is more acidic, and a pH above 7 is more alkaline.

At a pH of 5.5 and below the teeth begin to demineralize, putting them at risk for cavities. A healthy mouth is in a neutral pH range. For healthy teeth, keep oral acidity to a minimum. Teeth can remineralize and become stronger when the mouth has a pH of 7.0 or higher.

Chapter Three – Julia Roberts Smile

Julia Roberts attributes her bright smile and gleaming teeth to brushing with baking soda. She says as a young girl she watched her grandfather brushing his teeth with sodium bicarbonate, Baking Soda, putting a heaping glob on his toothbrush and scrubbing all around his teeth. He had only one cavity in his lifetime and advised her to use it.

Years ago the Arm and Hammer Baking Soda Company touted how baking soda could be used as a medicine. Today, sodium bicarbonate is used in many toothpastes. It is claimed that it is the very best agent for oral health because it alters the pH in the mouth interfering with bacteria production which have an adverse effect on oral health and even can cause adverse reactions in the body. It is thought that it can neutralize the acids in the oral bacteria.

Studies have revealed that bicarbonate inhibits plaque formation on teeth and increases calcium absorption by dental enamel.

Sodium Bicarbonate has the power to break through pathogen films that sticky stuff that turns into hard tarter.

The pH of sodium bicarbonate is 8.3, and the pH of saliva is 7.0. Sodium Bicarbonate should not be used for a couple hours after eating as it would neutralize the stomach acidity used in digesting foods.

One concern about sodium bicarbonate is its hardness. On a hardness scale it is 2.5 and dentin is 3-4. There could be concern that it could abrade dentin in a tooth. Dentin usually shows up at the gum line as enamel is abraded from the tooth. Hardness of tooth enamel is 5.0. Sodium Bicarbonate is widely used as a tooth brushing product so companies are willing to have people use it. If anyone is concerned about this, they should check with their dentist to see if using Sodium Bicarbonate is right for them.

In the world of tooth care, sodium bicarbonate is increasingly used in toothpastes and appears to be less abrasive to enamel and dentin than other toothpastes according to some reports. Check with your dental office for their opinion.

Chapter Four - Mouthwash

Using mouthwash regularly can improve your oral health. Most mouthwashes are acidic averaging 5.0 pH. Some people recommend staying away from alcohol based mouthwashes as there is concern about getting oral cancer from their use.

There are different types of mouthwashes – Anti-plaque, Whitening, Cosmetic, Antiseptic, and Fluoride. Ask your dentist what type of mouthwash is best for you.

Mouthwash needs to be swished around in the mouth for sixty seconds to be effective. Mouthwashes can help prevent cavities, slow the buildup of plaque, inhibit gum problems, and fight bad breath. Antibacterial products kill bacteria, or hinder their reproduction

Fluoride mouthwashes contain sodium fluoride which helps to strengthen the teeth as well as adding extra protection against tooth decay. However, fluoride is present in toothpaste and tap water. Too much fluoride is not healthy.

Antiseptic mouthwashes contain chlorhexidine gluconate - a chemical which inhibits the growth and reproduction of many microorganisms, including bacteria, as well as fungi, protozoa, and viruses. They are also helpful for people with bad breath.

My dentist uses Crest Pro Health mouthwash, and his office gives away samples of Listerine Cool Mint Antiseptic, Listerine Total Care Anticavity Mouthwash with .02% Sodium Fluoride, Listerine Zero Mouthwash with no alcohol, Listerine Zero Anticavity with .02% Sodium Fluoride with no alcohol.

Dentistry for Total Body Wellness lists the pH's of the following mouthwashes:

1. Listerine Total Care Mouthwash – 5.44
2. Listerine Antiseptic Mouthwash – 4.88
3. Listerine Zero Mouthwash – 6.02
4. Crest Pro Health Clinical Deep Clean – 5.18
5. Crest Pro Health - 4.27

Chapter Five - Regular Dental Checkups

To have good oral hygiene and oral health it is important to have regular dental checkups and cleaning of the teeth. It helps prevent gum disease.

A worst case scenario is to have an impacted tooth that can lead to blood poisoning and death. There have been reports that gum disease can cause strokes and heart attacks. Regular check-ups help preserve your teeth and make you feel better. Stains from smoking, tea, coffee can be removed, and cleaning helps prevent bad breath.

After your cleaning and checkup, you are leaving the office with gleaming white teeth and a brilliant smile.

Tooth enamel is mostly made up of minerals which accounts for its strength as well as brittleness. It ranks 5 on Mohs hardness scale. Dentin is 3-4 in hardness.

Sodium Bicarbonate (Baking Soda) hardness is 2.5 with an RDA (Relative Dentin Abrasivity) of 7. The dentin that is exposed on the tooth is mostly what is abraded by toothpastes and tooth powders.

RDA measures the erosive effect of abrasives on tooth dentin. Abrasivity of toothpastes are measured, and for FDA approval have to be under 200.

RDA Table

0 to 80	Low Abrasive
70 to 100	Low Range Abrasive
100 to 150	Highly Abrasive
150 to 200	Regarded as Harmful

It is reported that tooth whitening toothpastes appear to have more abrasivity than other toothpastes. The lower the RDA number the less abrasive is the toothpaste. Toothpastes range from eight to two hundred with one hundred being about the average of abrasivity. Toothpaste manufacturers regularly check the abrasivity of their toothpastes which is required by the FDA.

Chapter Seven - Brushing the Teeth

I use a Philips Sonicare Toothbrush that I purchased from my dentist's office which he recommended. Having always been a lousy tooth brusher this makes up for my inability to brush properly with a brush. I find it works wonderfully.

Tips from Philips Sonicare on Brushing

"Make sure you apply your brush head at the right angle.

You want to put the brush flat on the teeth for maximum contact, right? Nope. Placing the brush at a 45-degree angle against your teeth, pointing toward the gum line, is the proper form. This applies a hard, consistent edge against the teeth and acts like a broom that not only cleans your enamel but also keeps the gums fresh.

With an electric toothbrush like the Philips Sonicare Diamond Clean, all those discussed movements completely change. The brush itself does the quick brushing strokes employed up there (31,000 of them per minute, to be specific), so all you have to do is move it slowly and smoothly over every tooth, front and back, sweeping along the gum line.

Gums are not only the most neglected part of oral health, but they're one of the most important. Aside from the fact that the Philips Sonicare Diamond Clean promises healthier gums in general, our expert pointed out that the gum health setting offers a wider cycle movement to clean the gum pockets and keep them tough."

Chapter Eight - Brushing the Gums

Brushing the gums removes film and plaque bacteria that cause bad breath. Also, it stimulates the gums promoting blood flow into those tissues making them healthier.

For gingivitis, one unproven procedure is to make a paste of baking soda and water and massage around the gums for three minutes three times a week.

Oral Bacteria - It has been estimated that there are 20 billion oral microbes in the mouth.

Remineralization of Teeth

My dentist says that saliva has calcium ions and phosphorus ions that remineralize the teeth where cavities might be starting.

Chapter Nine - Manual Toothbrushes

The ADA Seal of Acceptance is recognized by dentists and consumers as the Gold Standard. When choosing toothbrushes, it would be a good idea to select one with the ADA Seal of Acceptance. The seal shows that a toothbrush is safe and effective at removing plaque.

The consensus recommendation for tooth brushes is to use soft bristles that cause minimal gingival abrasion. Most dentists recommend soft bristled toothbrushes. Soft bristles have a.15mm thickness.

For people with sensitive gums or teeth, an extra soft bristle should be used. Toothbrushes should be replaced every three to four months or when the bristles lose their firmness.

Chapter Ten - Should We Chew Gum?

The answer is yes unless chewing causes problems with your jaws. Consult with your dentist about this.

When chewing gum, the chewing and the artificial sweeteners increase the flow of saliva dramatically, which neutralizes acids in the mouth and washes away food particles on the teeth. Saliva has a 7.0 pH and neutralizes your mouth and has calcium ions and phosphate ions to remineralize surfaces on the teeth.

Clinical evidence shows that chewing gum with Xylitol reduces the formation of cavities. It has been shown that sugar free Xylitol gum stops the bacteria on the teeth from causing cavities. Recommendations about chewing Xylitol gum vary from two-to-three times a day to five-to-seven times a day. I chew three-to-five times a day. I find just after eating if I chew one or two sticks of Trident with Xylitol gum that my teeth feel cleaner and my mouth feels refreshed.

Chapter Eleven - Xylitol

What is Xylitol? Xylitol is a polyalcohol or sugar alcohol. Xylitol is made from Xylose and was originally made from birch bark, mushrooms, and raspberries. Xylose comes from a range of woody materials like straw and corn cobs.

It is reported that Xylitol causes cavities to remineralize by elevating the pH in the mouth and being a non-sugar the bacteria cannot feed on it, and they die off. It is claimed that Xylitol increases the flow of saliva which has calcium ions and phosphate ions which repairs cavities when the pH is 7 or above. Chewing gum also increases the flow of saliva It is said that Xylitol neutralizes the mouth. Saliva is a natural remedy for cavities with its calcium and phosphate content.

In Finland during WWII, sugar shortages resulted in Xylitol being used in its place which was made from birch trees that were plentiful in Finland. Years after the war the

Finns realized that the use of Xylitol had reduced cavities, and this was later proven by studies at the University of Turku. Over a hundred people were tested with sucrose, fructose, or xylitol. Those getting sucrose fared the worst followed by fructose, and those taking xylitol had no cavities.

In other studies, for testing, xylitol gum was used because it was easy to compute the dosage being given. Chewing xylitol once a day had little effect, three times a day reduced cavities by 60%, and five times a day reduced cavities by 80%.

Streptococcus Mutans is the main culprit in causing tooth decay, by causing plaque on the teeth. They take sugar from food and metabolize it and make acid in the process that eats through enamel on the teeth which is the start of a cavity. Xylitol inhibits this process.

Just a little while ago I went to the dentist for a cleaning and a check-up, and I had no cavities and no sign of any bleeding gums and little plaque. I could tell that the dental hygienist was like amazed as I have had bleeding gums forever. The last time I went to her I had some bleeding gums on my upper gums, and the time before that had problems on my upper and lower gums.

A little over three months before I began my routine of chewing Trident Xylitol gum, and after doing my regular brushing in the evening lightly brush around all my teeth with baking soda, and sometimes do some baking soda light brushing during the day. The baking soda reduces acidity in the mouth because it is 8.1 to 8.3 on a pH scale. Somewhere I read that baking soda knocks out gingivitis, and I read about one person who uses baking soda for gingivitis. How it is working for me I have no clue. So, the combination of using baking soda for brushing and chewing Trident Xylitol gum is clearly working for me In just over three months. Evidently, chewing Xylitol gum arrests the bacteria causing gingivitis as they cannot assimilate the alcohol sugars in Xylitol.

In a Healing Teeth Naturally article on www.Healingteethnaturally.com they cite a renowned dental researcher: "Dr. Paul H Keyes, D.D.S., clinical investigator at the National Institute of Dental Research, maintained that regular brushing with Salt and/or Baking Soda absolutely prevents all destructive periodontal (gum) disease, and said that he had never seen periodontal(gum) problems in patients who used salt or baking soda dentrifices(pastes) with any degree of regularly."

Chapter Thirteen - Rinsing the Mouth with Water

My father-in-law worked in big ticket at Sears on the sales floor with a guy who frequently rinsed his mouth with water from the water fountain during the course of the day to prevent cavities. My father-in-law said it seemed to work because this guy had very few fillings and never knew him to have any cavities.

This makes sense because rinsing with water would dilute and wash away acidity in the mouth which causes cavities plus helping to wash away food particles or debris on the teeth. Water with a pH of 7.0 would help neutralize the mouth which would inhibit cavities which develop in a 5.5 pH and below environment.

Chapter Fourteen - Choosing the Right Toothpaste

Check with your dentist to see what toothpaste is right for you. If you have sensitive teeth, a sensitive toothpaste is in order. More acidic toothpastes can be damaging to your enamel. Toothpastes with abrasives can abrade and damage the enamel. Fluoride is a weak base with a 6.6 pH that helps remineralize the teeth. Dentists recommend fluoridated toothpaste to reduce cavities.

My dentist gives me samples of Colgate Sensitive toothpaste and Colgate Total toothpaste to use. I have been using Colgate Total toothpaste for years.

Make sure you select a toothpaste that is approved by the American Dental Association.

Chapter Fifteen - Flossing

Flossing is an important oral hygiene practice. Tooth decay and gum disease can develop when plaque is allowed to build up on teeth and along the gum line. Professional cleaning, tooth brushing, and cleaning between teeth (flossing and the use of other tools such as interdental brushes) have been shown to disrupt and remove plaque.

The American Dental Association reports that flossing between the teeth is an integral part of oral health and is an important oral hygiene practice. Flossing and interdental brushes disrupt and remove plaque. Tooth decay and gum disease occur when plaque builds up on the teeth and along the gum line.

The American Dental Association recommends brushing the teeth for two minutes twice a day using a fluoride toothpaste.

The American Dental Association has ADA approved products that are marked with their acceptance symbol.

Here is the site for products that they approve:

http://www.ada.org/en/science-research/ada-sealof-acceptance/ada-seal

Chapter Sixteen - Fluoride

The American Dental Association recommends use of Fluoride Toothpaste. For children, check with your dentist for use of Fluoride Toothpastes. Ingestion of too much Fluoride can cause fluorosis.

Fluoride is a natural element that is also synthesized in laboratories and added to drinking water, toothpaste and mouthwash to prevent tooth decay. It protects teeth from the acid produced by bacteria in the mouth. The acid leads to demineralization and Fluoride remineralizes areas of tooth decay when the mineral adheres to the enamel.

Medical professionals recommend that adults and children consume fluoride daily to help prevent cavities. Fluoride may strengthen children's developing permanent teeth against decay. Some people oppose the fluoridation of water, citing the health concerns against fluoride and saying that there is insufficient evidence showing that it prevents tooth decay.

Laboratories produce fluoride. This type of fluoride is used by local water operators to fortify drinking water to prevent tooth decay in communities using the water. It is also added to consumer products, such as toothpaste and mouthwash.

Demineralization of teeth is combatted by the use of Fluoride. Bacteria found in the mouth combines with sugar to create acid. The acid causes erosion of tooth enamel.

Use of Fluoride leads to strengthening of tooth enamel, which is a known as remineralization.

There are varying levels of fluoride in some popular teas: black tea, white tea, green tea and oolong tea. *The fluoride content in some tea leaves can be high.*

My father grew up in Cambridge, Maryland where the water was naturally fluoridated and still is today. Aquifers deep under the Choptank River provided the fluoridated water supply.

My father had one cavity in his entire lifetime, and his brother Don is ninety-five years old and has had one cavity. My father always attributed his good teeth to the naturally fluoridated water in the Cambridge water supply. I contacted the Cambridge Municipal Water Authority and asked them about the Cambridge water supply. The water is naturally fluoridated from four wells which are mixed to Water Quality Standards.

I talked with a lady, an office manager at the water company, and asked her about cavities in Cambridge and how much fluoridation in the water supply contributed to dental health. I told her about my father growing up in Cambridge and having one cavity in his life time. She mentioned that she had cavities, and her daughters had cavities so she thought heredity had a lot to do with dental health.

How fluoride helps with preventing cavities from naturally fluoridated water seems to depend on the individual. For fluoridated water to help in preventing tooth decay, the process occurs when teeth are being formed in the mouth during childhood. It is said that there are 25% fewer cavities with fluoridated water.

Chapter Seventeen - Young Children

The American Dental Association now recommends starting babies on Fluoride Toothpaste with their first tooth. Be sure and check with your pediatrician and dentist and follow their guidelines for fluoride use.

ADA News Release: "CHICAGO, Feb. 10, 2014 —To fight cavities in children, the American Dental Association's Council on Scientific Affairs (CSA) is updating its guidance to caregivers that they should brush their <u>children's teeth</u> with fluoride toothpaste as soon as the first tooth comes in. This new guidance expands the use of fluoride toothpaste for young children.

To help prevent children's tooth decay, the CSA recommends that caregivers use a smear of fluoride toothpaste (or an amount about the size of a grain of rice) for children younger than three years old and a pea-size amount of fluoride toothpaste for children 3 to 6 years old.

Chapter Eighteen - Dr. OZ on Eating Crackers

Dr. OZ had a dentist on his show who said that eating crackers was the worst thing to eat because the cracker particles stick to the insides of the mouth as well as to the teeth.

Chapter Nineteen - Oral Health - Tongue Care

White coating on the tongue is an indication of bacteria and other build up on the tongue. The tongue should be a uniform pink color all over.

Bacteria on the tongue can be a cause of bad breath. Dentists recommend that the tongue be brushed as part of your brushing routine. Gently brush the tongue from back to front with your toothbrush.

During a routine check-up, dentists will usually check your tongue for any abnormalities.

It is also recommended to brush your gums gently, and the inside of your mouth gently.

Chapter Twenty - My Daily Brushing

First thing in the morning, I hand brush my teeth with a 7.35 pH toothpaste also brushing my tongue and gums after brushing my teeth, and then rinse my mouth with a 5.18 pH mouth wash for sixty seconds. Then, I use a hand toothbrush and put some baking soda, not a lot, on the bristles and lightly brush my teeth leaving baking soda in my mouth not spitting much if any out and not swallowing the baking soda. The idea being to create a more alkaline medium in my mouth with baking soda having a pH of 8.3.

During the day, after eating, sometimes I use a hand tooth brush and lightly brush my teeth and gums with baking soda to make my mouth more alkaline which also helps remove particles of food once again not swallowing the baking soda or spitting much if any out, and I do not

rinse my mouth out.

Acidity chart of Mouthwashes:

http://www.wellnessdentistrynetwork.com/uploads/article_files/wdn_14

56398362-1.pdf

Before going to bed, for sixty seconds I rinse with a

fluoride mouth wash with a pH of 5.18, and then brush my

teeth for two minutes with a Sonicare Electric Toothbrush

with a 7.35 pH toothpaste. Then, I use a hand toothbrush

or my Sonicare electric toothbrush with a little baking

soda on the bristles and brush lightly around all my teeth

to make a more alkaline medium in my mouth to make it

difficult for cavities to form. With cavities forming at a pH

of 5.5 and below and baking soda having a pH of 8.3 my

thinking is that this would make my mouth more alkaline

when I go to bed making an environment less conducive to

the formation of cavities. The whole idea of this brushing

process is to prevent cavities from forming and have a

healthy mouth and luxurious smile.

Chapter Twenty-One - Conclusion

Hopefully, some of this information about caring for the teeth and gums will be of value and will be helpful in eliminating some of the problems related to cavities and gum problems.

If you find some of this information worth trying that you haven't done before, the ultimate determination if it is helpful to you will be when you go to the dentist and the dentist tells you your mouth is a lot healthier, and I don't see any problems. Also, your mouth may tell you it is feeling better.

Careful brushing and cleaning the teeth and trying to maintain pH levels in the mouth at 7.0 and above would be extremely beneficial in reducing the acids that cause dental cavities. By all accounts, use of fluoride is recommended to help prevent cavities as well. To help reduce cavities, cut down on sugars and sweets in the diet. One can of Cola contains nine and a half teaspoons of sugar. Panera Bread reports that a twenty ounce cola fountain drink contains nine and a half teaspoons of sugar.

The goal of this book was to have No More Cavities. With all the foods we eat and the complex chemistries going on in the mouth with the varying pH's, completely eradicating cavities is an impossibility for most of the population.

What is possible is to have fewer cavities, better oral hygiene, cleaner teeth, feeling better, healthier gums, and brighter smiles.

My original thinking when I started this book was that pH was the key to controlling cavities and oral heath which turned out to be right. A pH of 5.5 and below is conducive to the formation of cavities. Eating a balanced diet, reducing sugar intake, and having a pH level around 7.0 except when eating in the oral cavity is the key to reducing cavities and having a healthy mouth and gums.

Acidic foods and acidic drinks lower the pH in the mouth particularly sugar as it clings to the teeth and bacteria feed on the sugar creating acids making the mouth more acidic. My thinking is that applying a thin coat of baking soda to the teeth after brushing the teeth and rinsing with mouth wash just prior to going to sleep will make the mouth more alkaline and less receptive to cavity and plaque formation while sleeping. It seems to work for me.

The End

www.ingramcontent.com/pod-product-compliance
Lightning Source LLC
Chambersburg PA
CBHW060817260726
48660CB00002B/1001